Acid Reflux Diet

—————— ❧❧❧❧ ——————

The most comprehensive diet to cure acid reflux

Kirsten Yang

TABLE OF CONTENT

Additionally, the information in the following pages is intended only for informational purposes and should thus be thought of as universal. As befitting its nature, it is presented without assurance regarding its prolonged validity or interim quality. Trademarks that are mentioned are done without written consent and can in no way be considered an endorsement from the trademark holder.

CHAPTER 1 :

WHAT IS ACID REFLUX?

Acid reflux disease has just come into the media spotlight recently. This is because of the development of different medications and treatments for acid reflux. In other words, because, drug companies can make some money from finding a cure for acid reflux, there seems to be a sudden outbreak of acid reflux disease.

Acid reflux disease explained in the easiest way possible is when you keep vomiting a little bit at a time. This not only does it put a terrible taste in your mouth, but it is also very uncomfortable.

Basically, you have stomach acid constantly being in your esophagus going up or going back down. Stomach acid is not meant to be in your esophagus for long periods of time and the acid eventually can greatly damage your esophagus which makes eating very difficult. You can also possibly get cancer of the esophagus, which is the worst possible scenario.

There are many causes for acid reflux and an explanation is needed on why so much stomach acid is in your esophagus and not in your stomach. Most of the time it is because of your lifestyle decisions that a person makes that cause acid reflux disease. If you are not exercising, not eating healthy or continue to smoke "cancer sticks" and drink alcohol you are a prime candidate for acid reflux disease.

CHAPTER 1 : WHAT IS ACID REFLUX?

Pregnancy can also cause acid reflux because the baby is pressing on your stomach. But at least you know this kind of acid reflux will eventually go away in 9 months or sooner. Unfortunately, the other kinds of acid reflux does not go away this easily and need to be addressed by a doctor. If you have heartburn or think you might have acid reflux, explained or unexplained, go see your doctor. The doctor can determine what kind of acid reflux you have and what the probable cause is and help get you the best treatment that you need.

Acid Reflux is very similar to heartburn, but acid reflux is a lot more uncomfortable than heartburn and definitely leads to a lot more potential health problem.

A quick way to find out if "it's just heartburn" is to take an over the counter heartburn relief medication. If you do not feel better from the medication and you can barely get a good night's sleep because of the acid burning in your throat you probably do have acid reflux disease.

Since acid reflux can now be explained there are a number of new medications that can help alleviate the problem. There are a lot of new prescription medications which many acid reflux sufferers are happy with and some that are not so pleased with.

Other alternatives include changing your sleeping position with special foam wedges and pillows to keep your body slightly inclined. This way the acid stays within its regular area of the stomach.

If you can learn some techniques for handling stress, especially if you get an upset stomach whenever you are upset or under pressure will help cure your acid reflux. Finally, watching what you eat and eating healthier can really go a long way in curing your acid reflux condition.

CHAPTER 2:

ACID REFLUX; THE CAUSE, AND THE SYMPTOMS

Not sure what that burning in your chest means? Two words that make your day a living nightmare, "Acid Reflux"! You have put up with the misery for maybe months and possibly years and it's time to do something about it! Acid Reflux or GERD (also called heartburn) affects millions of people each day and might be affecting you! The first step of action is to educate yourself on acid reflux and discover how you might naturally treat your heartburn.

THE CAUSE OF ACID REFLUX

There are numerous causes of Acid Reflux but knowing they could possibly allow you to find your problem. It might be a small habit you need to change or a drastic lifestyle makeover. Whatever the cause, it is necessary for you to take it seriously and make the adjustment quickly. The following is a list of causes for Acid Reflux:

1. Too much caffeine (coffee, tea, soda and chocolate) can cause Acid Reflux.

2. Consumption of alcohol (wine or beer) can cause Acid Reflux.

3. Smoking cigarettes can cause Acid Reflux.

4. Eating large meals can cause Acid Reflux.

5. Eating 2-3 hours before bedtime can cause Acid Reflux.

6. High-fat foods (especially fried foods) can cause Acid
   Reflux.

7. Foods containing tomatoes cause Acid Reflux.

8. Fruits and fruit juices cause Acid Reflux.

9. Tight fitting clothes around midsection can cause Acid
   Reflux.

THE SYMPTOMS OF ACID REFLUX

At its most basic, Gastroesophageal reflux disease (GERD), or
acid reflux, is a condition where the stomach backs up
(refluxes) and the acid within returns into the esophagus. If
you are wondering if you suffer from acid reflux, the following
are typical symptoms of Acid Reflux.

1. Heartburn (burning sensation ranging from the upper
   stomach to lower chest)

2. Regurgitation (food brought back up into the mouth)

3. Slight to Harsh Chest Pains

4. Difficulty in swallowing

5. Hoarseness in speaking

6. Dental erosion from stomach acids in mouth and throat

7. Asthma and/or a cough

CHAPTER 3:

THE GERD DIET

A cid reflux or Gastroesophageal Reflux disease (GERD) is a simple, yet sometimes a disease that can be both painful and chronic. The GERD diet is a part of a total treatment plan that includes both lifestyle changes and medication as well as dietary changes.

A diet plan is necessary to both reducing pain and allows healing in the affected areas of the esophagus. The changes in this specific diet include eating less and eating foods that are tolerated and thus eliminate the painful symptoms of acid reflux.

The GERD diet is only one part of an acid reflux treatment plan. A diet is used to prevent advancement of the disease and allow for healing in the affected organs. The diet consists of foods that are mild and do not cause a relaxation of pressure in the stomach, thereby opening the lower esophageal sphincter (LES).

The meals are lighter and eating before bedtime is eliminated. These are done in order to prevent acid reflux symptoms during the night. Before beginning a GERD diet plan you keep a food diary listing foods that are eaten, how much and all symptoms that are felt in addition to the severity of pain. This is used to determine what foods are causing the symptoms and what foods seem to help.

CHAPTER 3: THE GERD DIET

Chewing gum has been found to promote the continual production of saliva. This saliva has a high PH level and it is possible that it can promote a natural antacid effect upon the LES. Therefore, gum chewing on the GERD diet is encouraged whenever possible.

The diet, as stated above, makes use of the completed food diary and eliminates all foods that have previously caused acid reflux. In addition, with the GERD diet, it is recommended that all meals are lighter, especially in the evening hours before bedtime. This helps prevent nighttime occurrences.

Milk, previously thought by some to prevent acid reflux, has been shown to actually cause it when taken before bed. So drinking of milk before bed is prohibited. Alcohol is also prohibited as it has been known to cause acid reflux.

However, coffee, which previously had been automatically eliminated on the GERD diet is now allowed as tolerated, as it has been shown that not everyone is sensitive to coffee.

On the GERD diet other foods, also previously prohibited such as peppermint, spearmint, and chocolate, as well as hot and spicy foods, are also allowed as tolerated.

This is because the theory that milk cures ulcers and acid reflux and hot, spicy foods aggravate, it has been found to be somewhat of a myth. The GERD diet is one way you can get relief from your heartburn.

It is also an important aspect of acid reflux treatment and it is used to prevent severe complications of your GERD. So, be sure to follow your doctor or nutritionist's advice if they put you on a GERD diet.

CHAPTER 4:

SIMPLE STEPS TO HELP AGAINST GERD - ACID REFLUX DISEASE

There are many people who are being diagnosed with GERD. As strange as this may sound, GERD is commonly known as Acid Reflux Disease. I have a nephew who complained of nausea in the morning, stomach aches, and a sore throat.

After going to the doctor, he was diagnosed with gastroesophageal reflux disease, (GERD). This is a medical condition where the liquids from the stomach go back up into the esophagus.

The liquid contains stomach acids and can inflame and damage the lining of the esophagus. Fortunately, treatment is available for GERD. By changing your diet, taking the right types of medicines and modifying your sleeping habits, your GERD symptoms could diminish.

1. DIET

Certain foods can promote GERD. They reduce the amount of pressure in the lower esophageal muscle and cause the "reflux" to occur. Avoiding the following foods will help Chocolate, peppermint, alcohol, Fatty Foods, caffeinated drinks and even smoking.

CHAPTER 4: SIMPLE STEPS TO HELP AGAINST GERD - ACID REFLUX DISEASE

At meal time, try eating smaller meals earlier in the evening. The smaller meals will help keep the acids from going up the esophagus. By eating earlier, your stomach will have had a chance to fully digest your food.

Chewing gum can help reduce acid in the esophagus by increasing saliva production. Once swallowed, the saliva helps neutralizes acid in the esophagus.

2. TAKING THE RIGHT MEDICINES

Don't take plain old antacid tablets. These will only help for a very short time. There are two types of medicines on the market today specifically designed to help the symptoms of GERD. The first medicine developed specifically for the treatment of acid-related disorders was Tagamet. This product and others like it (Zantac, Axid & Pepcid) were designed to neutralize acids in the stomach.

Your stomach will continue to naturally produce acid, but these products will counteract that acid by neutralizing it. This type of medicine is best used 1/2 hour before a meal so it can get to work and be ready for the food digestion process.

These same medicines can be taken just before bed to help reduce the number of harmful acids being produced. Newer medicines have been created that work differently than these acid neutralizers just mentioned. Known as Proton Pump Inhibitors (PPI), these drugs actually block the production of antacids into the stomach.

Since the acid production is turned off, it will help prevent acid from going up the esophagus and promote healing from the burning and inflammation that is caused by Acid Reflux. Brands like Prilosec, Nexium, Protonix, and Prevacid are all PPI-type drugs and usually involve a doctor's script.

3. SLEEPING HABITS

Believe it or not, the way you sleep can promote GERD. Laying flat on your back allows the stomach acids to easily evacuate up into your esophagus. Elevate your bed where your head is positioned. Using a simple bed pillow to elevate your head won't help.

You need to elevate your upper body too. There are special wedge pillows available that are designed to do just this. For about 25 - 30 dollars you can sleep better at night. As always, consult your doctor about your health. Do not self-diagnose and always read the directions, warnings, and instructions on any medication you take.

The symptoms you are experiencing could be a more serious problem not related to GERD. Having said that, the simple changes to your diet, sleeping habits and the right medicines could significantly help your Acid Reflux Disease. Seek help and feel better.

CHAPTER 5:

ACID REFLUX RECIPES

When acid reflux becomes a regular part of life, the sufferer is commonly advised to change his or her diet. Try to avoid citrus, Try to avoid acids. See if the changes make it better. So you try. You experiment. And all the time, you're wishing there were acid reflux cure recipes. You finally go looking for such, and you find that there are cookbooks that focus on eating to avoid acid reflux.

The trouble is that neither you nor your doctor can say for sure that your current diet is the problem. You hate to put out money for an acid reflux cookbook only to learn that your acid reflux stems from another cause.

You'd like to find someone that inserts one little word in the phrase acid reflux cure recipes.

A. ACID REFLUX FREE CURE RECIPES

If you could just find acid reflux free cure recipes, you would try them. If it turned out that they did help, you wouldn't mind investing in one or two good acid reflux recipe cookbooks.

Acid reflux free cure recipes have three things in common.

1. They eliminate or reduce portions of those foods that are typically difficult to digest.

2. They include or increase portions of those foods that are known to aid in digestion.

3. They are FREE!

Orange juice, for example, is acidic. Many people claim that it increases acid reflux. So replace breakfast orange juice with a ripe banana, which is easy to digest. Or opt for an apple. Brownies and donuts are considered foods to be avoided by acid reflux sufferers.

They tend to sit, undigested, in the stomach. Choose an easily digested dessert such as a fat-free cookie or jelly beans.

ACID REFLUX RECIPE IDEAS

Here is a handful of ideas for acid reflux recipes.

1. Waldorf salad, made with ripe, healthy apples, nuts, and raisins, is a good acid reflux cure recipe. Use any traditional Waldorf salad recipe, but substitute low-fat mayonnaise and sour cream. You will have a great-tasting salad that contains no recognized acid reflux trigger foods.

2. Beef stew is another great acid reflux cure recipe. Use any beef stew recipe you like, omitting the onions. Cut the fat from the beef. If the stew seems to trigger acid reflux, eat a smaller portion next time.

3. Gingerbread is a marvelous dessert for acid reflux sufferers. Find a recipe that uses canned pumpkin and wheat germ. Make it with unsweetened applesauce and low-fat buttermilk. Then resist the temptation to mound whipped cream on top of it! Try a low-fat imitation whip instead.

4. Roast turkey breast is a good main course. Cranberries should be fine with it. Serve the potato, baked instead of mashed.

5. Lowly meatloaf is thought to have no specific acid reflux triggers.

6. Spaghetti may cause acid reflux in some. You can reduce the possibilities by beginning with acid-free tomato sauce. Omit garlic and onion from your sauce, and try using more basil and less oregano. There are a number of Italian spices that are great in spaghetti sauce. Try fennel with basil.

7. Cheesecake, too, can be an acid reflux cure recipe. Make it with reduced fat or no-fat cheeses. Use egg whites and/or egg substitute. While trying your acid reflux free cure recipes, learn what the actual cause of acid reflux is. You may be surprised to know that it is a muscular problem. There may be things you can do other than altering your diet.

Also for better understanding;

1. Consume food that is rich in complex carbohydrates

   Foods that are good for an acid reflux diet are foods that contain complex carbohydrates. Foods such as bread, pasta, and rice tend to absorb the acid and prevent it from backing up into the esophagus. Since these foods tend to put on weight, it is better to eat smaller portions of them. If you drink milk, switch to a milk that is lower in fat.

2. Stick to non-carbonated drinks

   Switch to drinks without carbonation. Decaf tea or coffee is a good choice but water is better. There are many flavored glasses of water that are quite good and good for you. Herbal tea is another good choice. You can experiment with the foods you eat to determine which foods cause you the most trouble. Everybody reacts to foods differently. By controlling your portions and eating high acid foods in moderation, you should be able to stick to an acid reflux diet without a lot of difficulties.

3. Use a nutritious meat

There are some excellent meats to include in this diet that is nutritious and delicious. Extra lean ground beef, steak, and chicken are usually great for the main course when on the best diet for acid reflux. Most fish is also very nutritious and safe for those with acid reflux. All of these are acceptable in the best diet for acid reflux, but these should not be cooked with a lot of greases. Those who want to avoid the symptoms of acid reflux might want to grill or broil the dishes.

4. Use wheat based food items

Most bread, cereal and graham crackers should not produce the symptoms of acid reflux. Cornbread and pretzels are good additions to the best diet fiber acid reflux. The best diet for acid reflux will eliminate some desserts, but other desserts should be fine for those with this condition.

5. Use cheese

Cheese often makes a good dessert, and there are some cheeses that will be an important part of the best diet for acid reflux. Fat-free cookies are usually fine for those with acid reflux. People with acid reflux should avoid rich, creamy cakes and most ice creams.

6. Use ginger

Gingers have some healing qualities, and those with acid reflux might try adding ginger to some of their food and beverages. Fresh ginger is available in the grocery stores, and this can be ground up and added to meals. Some dishes call for this in the recipe, but it can be added to other dishes. Ginger can also be added to tea. There are some cuisines that include ginger in many dishes such as Chinese cuisine. Those with acid reflux might patronize the Chinese restaurants and look for those dishes with ginger.

7. Drink tea

People with acid reflux should try to add green tea to their diet as this beverage is known to help the body digest other food and beverages. Herbal teas contain substances such as chamomile and licorice root provide a repair mechanism for the stomach so those with acid reflux should consume these teas if possible.

People with acid reflux should try to drink plenty of water, which will help the body excrete the excess acid more efficiently.

CHAPTER 6:

GUIDELINES ON PROPER ACID REFLUX DIETS AND FOOD TO AVOID

Before taking medication, most doctors will advise that the person with acid reflux disease make some changes to his/her diet, i.e. have a proper acid reflux diet plan. It is an easy and useful change that one can make. A proper diet for acid reflux could make a huge difference to the health and comfort of many people.

With a proper diet for acid reflux, it could remove all of the symptoms attributed to this condition and provide for a more undisturbed sleep. An effective and proper acid reflux diet plan includes knowing what food to avoid, what food to consume and good eating habits.

In this book, we shall go through some important guidelines that you can take away.

1. Avoid spicy food

    Stay away from spicy foods. Even foods you don't think taste spiciness can play a big role in creating acid reflux, so knowing what's in your food and knowing to stay away from food with spices in them is a great way to naturally remedy acid reflux. This isn't to say you are limited to nothing but bland foods now, it just means be as liberal as possible when eating spices that can irritate your stomach to the point of being in pain.

2. Cut down on large meals

    A recommended choice of acid reflux diet plan has always included eating several small meals every day instead of three large meals as what most people do. This is a good eating habit for everyone, even if you don't experience from acid reflux disease. This is to let the stomach to have sufficient capacity for proper digestion.

3. Avoid any meal just before bedtime

    Consuming just before bedtime, especially heavy meal, is prone to cause reflux problems. This is because the stomach has to produce great amounts of acid in order to digest the food.

    The excessive acid tends to back up into the esophagus when you lie down. Generally, a good practice is to eat your last meal before 8 pm daily.

4. Avoid fast foods

    Fast food is high in fat and will cause your stomach to produce more acid. Fast foods can also lead to weight gain, which will add to the problem of acid reflux.

5. Limit or avoid alcohol

    Alcohol will add to the secretion of acid in the stomach. It may also curb the contraction of the esophageal sphincter. It is the failure of the sphincter muscle to contract tightly that leads to acid reflux.

6. Avoid frying foods whenever possible

   Baked or broiled will serve two purposes; it will help control acid reflux symptoms and help to maintain a lower weight.

   Do not drink alcohol in excess, especially fruit wines. Having a small glass of wine with dinner will probably be OK, but keep it to a minimum of one to two times a week.

7. Avoid foods that stimulate acid production

   An acid reflux person should avoid foods that increase the secretion of acid in the stomach. These foods include coffee, spicy foods, tomatoes, citrus fruits, chocolate, and alcohol.

CHAPTER 7:

UNHEALTHY FOOD COMBINATIONS THAT YOU SHOULD AVOID IF YOU HAVE GERD (ACID REFLUX)

Many people would want to know how to naturally cure their GERD, acid reflux, or any digestive disorder they have. They may have been tired of taking the same medicines prescribed by their doctor again and again, and have not achieved significant results.

This is why many are now looking for alternative means to relieve and if possible cure their condition. One of the ways is to practice proper food combining in order to bring your digestive system to heal and repair itself from one's past mistakes; one's unhealthy eating habits.

There are actually unhealthy food combinations that you should avoid, but 3 of these standout and these are usually the typical diet of most individuals:

1. Hamburger and Fries: You read that right. Knowing this truth might cost the regular fast food restaurants around your area a lot of profits, but your health is the issue here. We all know how juicy a hamburger is and how good it is to go with the fries. However, the basic problem here is that one is a protein and the other a starch, and these two should never be combined with any meal at any given time.

If you are suffering from GERD, acid reflux or any stomach ailment, think about the time when you were regularly taking your doctor's medication and still feeling the same lame results. Could it be that you just couldn't resist this type of food?

2. Spaghetti and Meatballs: Aaah yes. I won't be having any hamburger and fries, so I'll just go for my second best favorite, spaghetti, and meatballs! Surely that won't be any problem, right? Unfortunately, the same can be said for this delectable food combination.

Spaghetti is mostly made up of starch (and sometimes the sauce itself can aggravate your GERD or acid reflux), and meatballs are a concentrated type of protein. It's hard to admit, but these two are not just compatible with each other, although I know, they admittedly taste good together.

3. Eggs and Toast: For those of you who like to have this as one of your meal combinations every breakfast time, think again. You're better off starting out the day with a choice of your favorite fruits (alone) than thinking that eggs and toast would give you that much-needed boost of energy you need to get going.

Again, one is a protein and the other a starch. All three food combinations are just that tasty and some are even mouth-watering. You may even be caught up in the habit of making any or all of these three a regular diet. But the fact remains, they are a recipe for digestive disaster.

Digestive problems such as GERD are the number 1 reason people visit their doctors today. The tragedy is most people spend their whole lifetime in treatment and traditional medication, only to feel the same, or a lot much worse.

Hey, I myself felt like a lab rat undergoing trial and error approaches by my doctors and gastroenterologists, while they kept on burning a hole in my wallet.

CHAPTER 8:

TREATMENT OPTIONS AVAILABLE FOR ACID REFLUX

A cid reflux treatment may differ from person to person, depending on the severity of the disease and the individual's body condition. Unfortunately, there isn't one fit of acid reflux cure for all. Acid reflux disease treatments can be classified into 5 main sections:

1. Changing your lifestyle as an acid reflux cure

In most acid reflux diseases, adopting lifestyle changes as a natural cure for acid reflux may be sufficient to control the pain and discomfort of acid reflux. The first step in treating acid reflux disease is to refrain from food that causes acid reflux. Other lifestyle changes include avoiding excessive eating, alcohol, coffee and smoking.

An overweight person may shed the excess pounds as a part of the acid reflux treatment plan. Since acid reflux symptoms can be worsened at night due to the lying position, raising the upper body by about eight inches while sleeping can give you a better sleep at night. Alternatively, you may choose to use an acid reflux pillow.

CHAPTER 8: TREATMENT OPTIONS AVAILABLE FOR ACID REFLUX

2. Over-the-counter acid reflux medicine

If lifestyle changes are not sufficient, you may have to resort to over-the-counter acid reflux medicine. Over the counter medications that are meant to treat acid reflux symptoms are common choices for millions of people daily. Products like Tums, Pepto Bismol, and Rolaids are convenient, cheap and don't require a doctor's prescription.

They function well in calming heartburn and other symptoms of acid reflux or indigestion. The widely available over-the-counter acid reflux medicines also included are antacids and H2 blockers. Antacids work on the principle of reducing the amount of acid in the stomach, whereas H2 blocker blocked the secretion of acid in the stomach.

When the acidity in the stomach is lessened, the occurrence of acid reflux reduces too. But, there are some harmful side effects that one should take note. Some of these are constipation or diarrhea, stomach cramps, or an increased thirst.

3. Prescribed acid reflux medication

In other chronic cases, a prescription acid reflux medication might be necessary. If medication is required for acid reflux treatment, it is likely that the acid reflux medication will have to be taken regularly and continued indefinitely.

These medications include prescribed version of H2 blocker and proton pump inhibitors.

4. Natural cure for acid reflux

The best natural remedy for acid reflux is still lifestyle changes as mentioned above.

Other natural cures may use herbal remedies for acid reflux such as herbal tea, cinnamon, pineapples, grapefruit and chicory root tea. Some people make use of homeopathic cure such as acid reflux and vinegar.

Eat bread, rice, and potatoes. These foods are always on the "do not eat" list because of their high carbohydrate count, but these foods do wonders for soaking up acidic fluids in your stomach.

This method doesn't require you to overeat carbs, but by having even one piece of bread, a half cup of rice or half a potato during a full meal, you can dramatically decrease the amount of acid reflux you experience after eating. One should always proceed with caution when using another acid reflux medicine.

ACID REFLUX SURGERY

For those who do not wish to depend on medication indefinitely, or the medication is simply ineffective, the last option is acid reflux surgery. Acid reflux surgery involves a laparoscopic procedure to wrap and suture the upper part of the stomach around the esophagus.

There is a small video camera on the end of a thin tube. This camera is inserted through a small incision in the belly button. The abdomen is filled with carbon dioxide to inflate it so that the surgeon can see.

The camera allows the surgeon to see the instruments. This puts the right amount of pressure on the lower esophageal sphincter. Patients are often discharged the same day as the surgery.

This is an easy, straightforward procedure that can relieve the pain of acid reflux. Recovery is generally quick and such surgery has a good track record of successful cases. Acid reflux surgery is considered only when other options are exhausted.

CHAPTER 8: TREATMENT OPTIONS AVAILABLE FOR ACID REFLUX

In many cases, it is necessary to avoid further complications of acid reflux. Once surgery has been performed, it is a good idea to stick to a healthy eating plan that cuts out those foods that cause acid reflux. It would be a shame to counteract the effectiveness of the acid reflux surgery.

Basically, searching for the right cure for your acid reflux is an about knowing your symptoms and how they come together in your body and affect your system. When searching for the right acid reflux treatment, you should always think of the long term effect.

Never go for the short term relief and overlook about the long term implication.

CHAPTER 9:

NATURAL REMEDIES FOR ACID REFLUX

Because prescription medications can sometimes have unwanted side effects, many people look for natural cures for acid reflux. In addition, most prescription medications were not designed to be taken for long periods of time, possibly while a person makes dietary and lifestyle changes which can be natural remedies for acid reflux.

Herbal remedies for acid reflux are based on what herbalists know of traditional medicine and traditional medicinal plants. Some of these are common food, herbs, which pose no danger for long-term use, but their effectiveness as natural cures for acid reflux has not been proven.

If you have been diagnosed with acid reflux, it is important to see your doctor regularly, even if you feel that your symptoms are under control. And you should let your doctor know about any botanical or herbal remedies for acid reflux that you may be using.

It is important to see your doctor regularly because stomach acid can damage the esophagus and lead to more serious conditions including cancer of the esophagus. If you are relying on natural cures for acid reflux and you become hoarse in the morning, develop a cough, or feel a need to clear your throat frequently, these may be symptoms of silent acid reflux.

Silent acid reflux is the term used to describe acid reflux that affects the voice box and the vocal cords but does not cause heartburn symptoms. So even if natural remedies for acid reflux keep your heartburn under control, you should still see your doctor regularly and report new or different symptoms.

Herbal remedies for acid reflux include chamomile, meadowsweet, slippery elm, cancer bush, fennel, catnip, angelica root, gentian root, ginger root and other botanicals, including aloe.

Slippery elm was used historically by native peoples to treat stomach upset, diarrhea, constipation, heartburn and other digestive complaints. Fennel and ginger root were also common "folk remedies" for the relief of indigestion. Modern herbalists have found that a combination of several of the herbs that had been used for indigestion could be effective natural remedies for acid reflux.

Some may call them natural "cures" for acid reflux, but the long-term relief of acid reflux is best accomplished by changes in lifestyle and eating habits.

For example, smoking relaxes the sphincter muscles that normally prevent stomach acid from reaching the esophagus. It also dries out saliva in the mouth and throat, which normally would neutralize some of the stomach acids and begin the digestive process.

If you use herbal remedies for acid reflux and you do not stop using tobacco products, then you may still have acid reflux and you are still at risk of developing esophageal cancer. The major risk factors for developing esophageal cancer include acid reflux, smoking, and alcoholism. This brings up another lifestyle change that is recommended for long-term control and relief of acid reflux.

Reducing or eliminating alcohol consumption can reduce acid reflux. In particular, alcohol consumption in the evening is believed to lead to more symptoms of nighttime acid reflux, as well as other health problems. While some argue that a glass of red wine has many health benefits, this is a 4-ounce glass, before a meal, and for those who suffer from acid reflux, even this may be a problem.

Alcohol increases stomach acid. Prescription and natural remedies for acid reflux are geared towards reducing or preventing excess stomach acid. It just does not make sense to continue to drink alcohol when you have been diagnosed with acid reflux.

Changing your eating habits may be natural cures for acid reflux. If you normally eat a large meal late in the evening, less than three hours before bedtime, then you are more likely to suffer from nighttime heartburn or other acid reflux symptoms like coughing.

This is because acid is traveling up out of the stomach and into the throat. Raising the head of the bed is also considered one of the natural remedies for acid reflux symptoms that occur at night. Gravity helps keep the acid in the stomach, but eating your last meal earlier and making it a smaller meal may prevent nighttime acid reflux.

Finally, weight loss should be mentioned as one of the natural cures for acid reflux. If you are currently at your ideal weight, then you may not need to read this section.

Overweight and obese people are much more likely to suffer from acid reflux, including nighttime acid reflux.

Trying herbal remedies for acid reflux control and making no effort to lose the extra pounds will undoubtedly be disappointing. Using prescription and/or natural remedies for acid reflux while you are trying to lose weight makes sense.

Avoiding fried and fatty foods are often recommended for people who suffer acid reflux.

CHAPTER 9: NATURAL REMEDIES FOR ACID REFLUX

If you avoid these and eat several small meals during the day, then you may naturally lose weight and naturally cure acid reflux.

Eating several small meals every couple of hours is often recommended by diet doctors, because it increases your metabolism and keeps blood sugar levels stable, so you don't feel sleepy after a meal, don't feel a need to lie down and stomach acid is less likely to travel back up into the esophagus.

CHAPTER 10:

WAYS TO RELIEVE ACID REFLUX

The condition of acid reflux is also commonly known as heartburn. This is a condition that is characterized by the inflammation of the esophagus, caused by the backing up of food from the stomach into the esophagus. This food is partially or mostly digested and usually has a high acidic content, which causes pain and/or discomfort in many people.

Several treatments have been used successfully in the fight against heartburn (acid reflux). Some of these forms of treatment include one or more of the following:

1. Baking soda and water: Usually a teaspoon of baking soda mixed in a glass of water will help most people since it neutralizes excess acidity. This is one of the most natural ways to cure heartburn/acid reflux.

2. Alka-Seltzer: This is a tablet that dissolves in water that is taken orally as a liquid. This product has a similar effect as baking soda and water. It can be purchased at a pharmacy or grocery store without a prescription.

3. Pepto-Bismol: This is a liquid medication that is taken orally to help alleviate the effects of heartburn. This is available without a prescription.

4. Clear Soda (such as Sprite or 7-UP): The carbonation in clear sodas can help to relieve the acid buildup in a person's stomach and can also help a person to release gas.

5. Tums: These are tablets that come in a chewable form which contains calcium carbonate, an ingredient that helps relieve symptoms of upset stomach and heartburn. It is termed an antacid.

6. Prescription Medications: Those who need relief from chronic heartburn (acid reflux) can consult a doctor or other qualified healthcare professional. They may prescribe more potent or different medications than those sold over-the-counter in stores. They will also provide instructions on how to take these.

7. Exercise: Those who engage in regular exercise will also find relief from heartburn in many cases. Usually, it is good to do a variety of aerobic and anaerobic movements.

   Examples of anaerobic exercise involve fast-paced step exercises and dance movements, as well as jogging, stair climbing, and bicycling. Types of anaerobic exercise include weight and resistance training and stretching exercises.

   More information can be found on specific exercise programs that can help people.

8. Diet Changes: If heartburn sufferers want relief, they may need to alter their diets.

9. Heat or Feet Pillows: Heartburn sufferers can also prevent or relieve acid reflux, particularly at night, if they raise their head or feet with pillows or another object (Such as a bed wedge).

   Propping up the head usually works best since gravity can help keep food from creeping upward into the esophageal area.

10. Relaxation: If people take the time to rest and relax, they are better able to reduce the amount of stress that could lead to poor choices.

    For example, it could reduce a person's desire to consume large amounts of alcohol, which can certainly aggravate the pain and discomfort associated with heartburn.

CHAPTER 11:

TASTY RECIPES FOR PEOPLE WITH ACID REFLUX (GERD) FOR ORDINARY DAYS

Bad eating habit is the key ingredient in the recipe for acid reflux. An unhealthy eating lifestyle will most surely lead to acid reflux disease. Technically, acid reflux is known as Gastroesophageal reflux disease (GERD).

Acid reflux happens when excess gastric fluid or partially digested food backflow into the food pipe. Some common symptoms of acid reflux disease are chest pains and heartburn, where the sufferer experiences a burning sensation in the chest and throat.

Other symptoms include vomiting and sleeplessness. To ensure that you're eating habits do not contribute to the acid reflux recipe, there are a few simple rules to follow. First and foremost, do not consume too much in one meal. Eating too much causes the stomach to produce more gastric food.

It would be good if you could break food intake into five or six small meals a day instead of three huge meals. Do not eat two hours prior to bedtime.

If you really must, then have a small snack two to three hours before bedtime. This will give your stomach time to digest the food before you go to bed.

CHAPTER 11: TASTY RECIPES FOR PEOPLE WITH ACID REFLUX (GERD) FOR ORDINARY DAYS

Next is to create an acid reflux diet. Like all food diet, there are the "good" foodstuff and the "bad" foodstuff.

Fresh fruits and vegetables will come under the "good food" list. However, it is advisable to avoid citrus fruits or juices as these may stimulate acid production in your stomach. Have some carbohydrates in your diet so that the gastric juices have something to work on. Observe moderation in each variety of food.

Avoid fatty meat, alcoholic drinks, drinks containing caffeine and carbonated soft drinks. All these "bad" foodstuffs are acid-stimulating. There are also other tips on reducing acid reflux, varying from sleeping position to posture and clothing. For example, it is believed that sleeping with the head slightly raised helps to keep the stomach juices from back-flowing into the esophagus.

The body of every human being reacts to different substances differently.

So make sure you consult your doctor and draw up an acid reflux disease prevention recipe that is ideal for your well-being.

1. ACID REFLUX BANANA TREATMENT

There are different ways to treat acid reflux symptoms, regardless of the cause. While some treatments involve the use of medications, other treatments take a more natural approach such as the acid reflux banana treatment.

Aside from being a really tasty and nutritious fruit high in vitamins and minerals, bananas contain virtually no fat, sodium, or cholesterol. For this reason, bananas are not only an integral part of a healthy diet, they can be used as a natural remedy to treat and prevent a number of health issues including, insomnia, depression, anemia, hypertension, and heartburn.

How exactly can a banana help with heartburn? Bananas have a natural antacid effect on the body. They primarily suppress acid secretion in the stomach by coating and protecting the stomach from acid, which helps against the formation of stomach ulcers and ulcer damage.

There are two ways in which the antacid property of a banana helps suppress acid:

Firstly, bananas contain a substance that encourages the activation of the cells that make up the lining of the stomach. As a result, a thicker mucus barrier is formed to provide the stomach with more protection against acid.

Secondly, bananas feature compounds called "protease inhibitors", which help to eliminate certain bacteria within the stomach that have been found to contribute to the development of stomach ulcers.

How can I add bananas to my diet? If you would like to help prevent heartburn by incorporating bananas, try eating a banana a half-hour before a meal, or directly after a meal. Some GERD (gastroesophageal reflux disease) sufferers also find eating a banana during a meal or half a banana before and after a meal beneficial. It's also a good idea to eat a banana when heartburn symptoms appear.

If the idea of eating a plain banana doesn't thrill you, there are more fun and tasty ways you can add bananas to your diet.

The following are some suggestions:

- Eat dried banana or mashed banana as a snack

- Cut up a fresh banana or use dried banana pieces and add it to cereal, yogurt, and salads

- Make a banana smoothie with live cultured yogurt

- Banana shakes (if you are allergic to milk and milk products, substitute with soy milk)

- Banana split - go easy on the ice cream

- Banana bread

- Banana muffins

- Banana cake

- Fruit bowl (excluding citrus fruits)

- Banana sandwich with cinnamon

Here are a few other facts to keep in mind when making banana recipes:

- Bananas with green tips are best used for cooking or should be left to ripen before eating.

- Bananas with yellow tips are best for eating

- Bananas that are browning or have dark brown or black specks are ideal for baking (Note: the riper the banana, the sweeter it will be because the starch has turned to sugar, making it better for baking)

- Bananas are the most popular fruit in America, are available all year round, and are low in cost, so it shouldn't be too difficult for you to make acid reflux banana remedies part of your regular diet. However, it is important that you eat bananas, according to your lifestyle requires. Keep in mind that Bananas are high in sugar.

Thus, if you are eating more than one banana per day, you do need to burn off the energy you are providing your body for maintaining a healthy body weight. Also, refrain from eating bananas close to bedtime because acid reflux can still occur when you are sleeping as the lower esophagus sphincter relaxes.

2. JUICER RECIPES

Juicing is a great way to make your diet healthier, and there are general rules you should follow to create your very own juicer recipes for energy. Juicing can be used to get the essential vitamins and minerals contained within fruits and vegetables without needing to actually fill up by eating them.

This book contains information about the beneficial effects of juicing and will guide you on how to create your very own juice.

If you want a healthy juice, choose a dark green vegetable for the base of your juice. You will want the juice to be between 50 to 75 percent spinach, chard, chard or something similar and make it at least half of what your juice is composed of.

This is what makes a "green smoothie" different from just a regular smoothie. These are the most effective ingredients for people who want to drink juice for health. Juices made exclusively from fruit often have more sugar and fewer nutrients than greens-based juices.

They can lend a bitter flavor to juice, however, so use them in conjunction with sweeter fruits or veggies, such as carrots, berries, and citrus. Fill the rest with your choice of fruits in order to achieve great taste. A popular berry blend is cranberries, blueberries, strawberries, and blueberries.

When you are juicing apples, use the ripest and sweetest apples that you can. If you decide to use bruised apples, make sure to cut the bruise off. Be creative and blend your own great-tasting juices.

CHAPTER 11: TASTY RECIPES FOR PEOPLE WITH ACID REFLUX (GERD) FOR ORDINARY DAYS

After you're done juicing, immediately wash all the equipment that you used. Each of the fruits and vegetables contains different vitamins and nutrients. Wherever possible, make sure that you get the right nutrients while also making sure that you are able to enjoy a tasty drink.

Use cranberries as part of your juicing routine if you are having any bladder condition or urinary tract infection. Start adding them the moment you start to feel symptoms of a problem.

Pay attention to the cues your body's signals concerning the juices you consume. You may drink something that your system doesn't like. If you drink a new juice and feel queasy or experience stomach churning, think about new fruits or vegetables you used in order to find the culprit. You can then use smaller amounts and condition your body to adjust to them.

Ginger is an all-natural remedy for soothing gastrointestinal issues. Ginger has many anti-inflammatory properties and can help with stomach ulcers and acid reflux disease or peptic ulcer disease.

If you are beginning to feel old and achy all the time, consider juicing as a great add-on to your life for a nice boost of energy! Juice offers several nutrients that may help assist your memory, aid memory or even slow down cell death due to free radicals.

As we said before, juicing is very good for you. When you juice, you get all the vitamins and minerals that are found in vegetables and fruits, but without the filling pulp.

By applying what you have learned in this article, you will be well on your way to juicing up your health. If you follow these principles, you will be well on your way to making your own delicious juice recipes for energy.

CHAPTER 12:

GREAT HERBS FOR ACID REFLUX

Taking herbs for acid reflux may be a beneficial way to avoid heartburn so you don't ever have to worry about confusing heartburn symptoms with a heart attack. Herbs can help you stop heartburn before it starts which will help you limit the number of antacids or other medications you may take for heartburn relief.

There are various herbs used as health remedies, but only some are truly effective at preventing and relieving acid reflux. The following are 5 effective herbs for acid reflux.

1. Black Pepper: This is an aromatic herb that enhances taste, improves gastric circulation, and stimulates digestion. Black pepper can be added to recipes or can be an additional feature to prepared meal. For best results, use a small (approximately a tsp.) amount of fresh black pepper whole and grind it over food.

2. Indian long pepper: Indian long pepper is a powerful stimulant for digestion and is one of the most recommended for enhancing digestion, assimilation, and metabolism of foods ingested. In addition, Indian long peppers are fantastic herbs for acid reflux disease,

as studies have found it can provide considerable protection against the development of gastric ulcers.

Indian long pepper should be taken in small amounts (approximately a tsp.), and can be purchased dry and used in recipes, or added to meals for flavor. Simply crush the pepper to add it to food. Keep in mind that if you use too much, the flavor can become too intense, and you may find it too hot to eat.

3. Ginger: Ginger has been used for thousands of years to aid in digestion and treat stomach distress such as nausea, vomiting, and diarrhea. Ginger is one of the most highly effective herbs for acid reflux, and it is likely the purest. The effectiveness of ginger is due to its anti-inflammatory, antimicrobial and analgesic properties. Fresh ginger root can be added to recipes or added as an extra garnish to a finished meal. Ginger can also be taken in powder form and in tea.

   Ginger is considered to be one of the safest herbal remedies to take, and you can ingest moderate amounts of it daily (I.E. tsp. of powder ginger, or an inch of a ginger root). However, be advised that if taken excessively, it may lead to mild heartburn.

4. Liquorice: Liquorice is a powerful herb and anti-inflammatory that studies have found are showing much promise as inhibiting the development of ulcers, wounds on the mucous membrane, and gastritis. Liquorice also acts like an antacid. Liquorice was also found to improve the secretory status of Brunner's gland, which is located throughout the duodenum system.

Brunner's gland works to protect against the development of duodenal ulcers. Liquorice is available in powder form and can be taken in tea. A cup of tea or 3 tsp. of powder liquorice daily is considered safe to take. High doses of liquorice can lead to symptoms such as a headache, water retention, and high blood pressure.

5. Indian gooseberry: Indian gooseberry is a fruit that has been used to treat peptic ulcers and ingestion that is non-ulcer related. Studies have found Indian gooseberry to have considerable antioxidant effects, and it significantly reduced gastric mucosal injury and acid secretion. Indian gooseberry is made up of cell-protective properties as well as anti-ulcer, and anti-secretory properties.

You can eat an Indian gooseberry raw with a little salt, or you can take it in powder form and in the form of tea. This herb is not associated with side effects, but should still be ingested in moderation, as it can act as a laxative if eaten in copious amounts.

When considering herbs for acid reflux, keep in mind that you shouldn't take herbs as a form of medicinal treatment without first consulting your doctor about your plans. This is because some herbs may interact with other herbs, with medications you may currently be taking, or other health conditions you may have.

CHAPTER 13:

TASTY ACID REFLUX RECIPES FOR 1 OR 2 WEEKS MUST READ

Curing oneself of the condition called acid reflux can be accomplished by using natural, healthy methods for some weeks. After a great deal of research I discover that with the proper use of herbs, health store items, meditation, exercise, and diet, one can heal themselves of acid reflux.

The first thing that I learned is that acid reflux, sometimes called GERD (gastroesophageal reflux disease), is not a disease at all. Contrary to what the medical community would have us believe, it is simply a condition, brought on by poor eating habits. Besides eating the wrong foods, not chewing food properly is probably the root cause of this ailment.

The Acid reflux condition would not exist without a damaged esophagus and a weakened LES (lower esophageal sphincter). If the condition is to be eliminated, healing the esophagus must be the first order of business. During this reflux recovery period, eating anything which could irritate or damage the esophagus, must be avoided.

Things like poorly chewed chips, crackers, cereal, or any hard foods with sharp edges are culinary culprits - they cause little lacerations to develop in the esophagus. Until the lacerations have had a chance to heal, spicy foods, such as acidic tomato products, hot peppers, raw garlic and raw onions should also be eliminated from the diet.

They just further irritate the condition. Smoking and drinking alcohol relax the LES, allowing stomach acid to splash up into the esophagus, thus impeding the healing process. The key to acid reflux recovery is to eat only mild, easy to digest food until the esophagus has healed.

Eat early, giving yourself at least three hours of sitting or walking time before lying down. Eat slowly and chew your food completely. And last, but not least, try to eat in a relaxed, pleasant environment.

I have listed a few of my favorite recipes that I enjoyed during my own recovery period. They can be made quickly and easily. Try doubling these recipes so that you can reheat them later in the week; less time in the kitchen.

Remember that cooking from scratch, instead of relying on convenience foods, is a better approach to good health, in general. It is also nice to know what you are really eating. For breakfast, I believe that fresh fruit is the best way to go. I especially like melon and papaya.

For lunch, I eat more fruit like apples, bananas and, perhaps, some almonds, or walnuts. It's better to eat many little healthy meals during the day. I try to buy only organic fruits, however, sometimes when I am rushed, I purchase "ready to go" containers of mixed fruit at the grocery store. Try to stay away from pineapple, as I find it hard to digest.

How about starters in the evening? Serving vegetables raw is the ultimate healthy way to present them. Try creating a beautiful platter of crudité (crew di tay) better known as elegant rabbit food. Serve it with a savory tofu dip. Use cauliflower, broccoli, English cucumbers, radishes, green & yellow zucchinis, Belgium endive, carrot sticks, whole small mushrooms, or whatever appeals to you. Cut the vegetables into bite size pieces for dipping.

The Belgium endive is a natural, edible scoop for dipping. Just cut off the ends and peel off the leaves. Make the tofu dip by putting one package of soft or silken tofu in a food processor or blender, adding garlic powder, cumin, paprika and chopped chives or parsley for flavor and color. Season with salt & pepper to taste.

Add a little fresh squeezed lemon juice if the mixture is too thick. Process until smooth and creamy. If you are in a rush, ready made dips and raw vegetable platters are available in the produce sections of most supermarkets, but make a concerted effort to eat only organic, if possible.

I hope that you enjoy the following dishes. Even though I have cured myself of acid reflux, I still cook these recipes on a regular basis. I prefer food slightly undercooked. Feel free to adjust the cooking times and seasonings to your own taste. Bon appetite!

SAUTÉED WHITE FISH ON A BED OF MASHED POTATOES

This recipe is for one serving. Increase the ingredients for additional servings as needed.

- One 4oz filet of white fish (orange roughy, sole, turbot, flounder, etc)

- One med. Potato

- Steamed green vegetable such as broccoli, spinach, peas or asparagus

- Parsley or chives for garnish

- ¼ tbsp unsalted butter, olive oil or Pam

We will start with the potatoes because they take the longest to cook and they tend to retain their heat the longest. The fish and vegetable take only minutes to cook.

Peel and cube potato. Place in cold water to cover. Bring to the boil, and then simmer until fork tender. Drain, leaving just enough cooking liquid for mashing or whipping. You may also use the vegetable broth (recipe below) instead. Add salt to taste. Hold in a warm place.

Season fish with salt and pepper to taste. Place non-stick sauté pan over med high heat. Add butter, oil or spray with Pam. When not quite smoking, add fish. Cook two minutes, turn and cook other side for two minutes, or until the filet is lightly brown and cooked through. If the file is very thin, one minute on each side may be enough. (You can broil or bake the fish if desired)

Serve fish on top of mashed potatoes, surrounded by the steamed vegetables. Garnish with chopped parsley or chives.

VEGETABLE BROTH

This broth is very alkaline and rich in minerals. It can be served as a simple soup or used as a stock (as above) for cooking. Cook and save the potatoes and beets, use as a vegetable side dish or to add to soup.

- 2 cups red-skinned potato peelings

- 3 cups celery stalk

- 2 cup celery tops

- 2 cups beet tops

- 1 small zucchini or yellow squash

- 2 cups carrots

- One small onion

- Sprig of parsley

- 2 ½ quarts distilled water

Chop all vegetables into very fine pieces. Place in water and bring to the boil. Simmer for 20 minutes. Strain & refrigerate for future use.

Note: By cooking pearled barley in the finished broth with the addition of chopped vegetables, one can prepare a healthy soup for a first course.

PASTA PRIMAVERA

Primavera means "spring" in Italian. This pasta dish offers a great opportunity to use all the wonderful fresh spring vegetables at your disposal. However, you can make this dish anytime of the year by using whatever fresh vegetables you can find at your food market.

I have chosen a mixture of vegetables that I happen to love, for this recipe. You can use these or replace them with your favorites. During the reflux healing period, try to stay away from tomatoes, raw onions and raw garlic. I

have included garlic in this recipe (*see note regarding roasted garlic). If you can tolerate a little garlic, then make sure to cook it well at a low temperature, without browning it.

If you want to be a bit daring, you can add the optional cup of heavy cream. You may substitute parsley for the basil and the penne regatta for fettuccine, or other pasta. The whole family can enjoy this

Classic pasta dish.

- 1 cup sliced mushrooms

- 1 cup sliced carrots

- 1 cup baby peas

- 1 cup sliced asparagus spears

- 1 cup snow peas or sugar snaps

- 2 cloves garlic, finely chopped or roasted

- 1 lbs. Penne Regatta

- 1 tsp. Salt

- 3 tbsp extra virgin, first cold pressed olive oil

- ½ cup shredded basil

- ½ cup Parmigiano-Reggiano cheese

- ½ cup heavy cream (optional)

Place a steamer basket in a pot with a small amount of water and bring to the boil. Place vegetables in a basket, cover, and steam until tender (about 4 minutes). Rinse under cold running water to stop the cooking and preserve the color, and drain. To a large pot of boiling water, add salt and the penne regatta. Cook uncovered according to the instructions on the box, preferably al dente. Meanwhile, in a large sauté pan, heat the olive oil. Add the garlic and cook on a low flame for a couple of minutes (do not brown). Add the steamed vegetables and optional heavy cream and raise the heat to medium. Cook just enough to heat.

Drain the pasta and add to the sauté pan and mix well.

Sprinkle with Parmigianino Reggiano, and shredded basil. Heat the dish thoroughly and serve. If the dish needs more salt, use extra cheese instead, at the table. Serve this dish with a heart of romaine salad with lemon chive dressing (recipe below)

* Note: It takes more than two cloves of roasted garlic, for this recipe. On a sheet of aluminum foil, place two heads of garlic and cut the stem end off with a knife. Drizzle a little olive oil over them and wrap tightly. Bake in a 400-degree oven for one hour.

When cool enough to handle, squeeze out the roasted garlic, into a bowl, discarding the shells. Mash well with a fork.

Another use for roasted garlic is my version of pesto sauce. I use walnuts instead of pine nuts, which I find indigestible, with the roasted garlic and basil. Use whatever proportion you like and drizzle first pressed, extra virgin olive oil into the blender. If your sauce is too thin, adjust with more walnuts, basil, and garlic. If it is too thick, use more olive oil. This is all a matter of taste. Serve with your favorite pasta. I prefer linguini or fettuccini.

LEMON CHIVE SALAD DRESSING

This is a simple, yet classic vinaigrette for green salads. Use heart of Romaine, Boston or Bipp lettuce. Make this dressing and hour or so before serving, in order that the chive flavor is fully incorporated. Remember to toss well before serving. The advantage here is using lemon juice, instead of vinegar. I find that lemon juice becomes alkaline after being ingested.

- 1 lemon juice

- Sea salt (pinch)

- 3 tbsp. extra fine sugar

- 6 tbsp. extra-virgin olive oil

- 6 tbsp. minced chives (you can't have too many)

FRESHLY GROUND BLACK PEPPER

Combine lemon juice, salt, and sugar in a mixing bowl. Whisk until the sugar and salt are dissolved. Continue whisking in the olive oil, chives and several grinds of pepper. Keep whisking until dressing is emulsified. (Note: You can make this dressing for two by reducing the lemon juice to two tbsp, and the other ingredients by 1/3.) Keep leftover dressing in a jar in the fridge for future use. It will keep for about a week.

SAVORY LENTILS WITH TEXMATI BROWN RICE

- 1 lb of organic lentils (2 ½ cups), rinsed

- 8 cups water or stock

- 1 onion, chopped

- 3 cloves of garlic, chopped

- 2 carrots, sliced

- 2 stalks celery, chopped

- 1 bay leaf

- 2 sprigs of thyme or ½ tsp dried

- Organic Texmati brown rice (follow instructions on package)

In a large pot, bring water and lentils to a boil. Add other ingredients. Reduce to the simmer, partially covered. Cook until tender (about 20 to 30 minutes), stirring occasionally and adding more liquid as needed. Remove the bay leaf and thyme sprigs. Season with salt and freshly ground black pepper to taste. Serve over organic Texmati brown rice. Garnish with chopped parsley. Serve with a light green salad, dressed with the lemon-chive dressing above.

BAKED CHICKEN BREASTS ON MUSHROOM CAPS WITH STEAMED BROCCOLI AND NEW POTATOES

- 6 chicken breasts (either bone in or halves with skin on)

- 1 tsp dried thyme

- Olive oil

- 6 large Portobello mushrooms (or enough smaller mushrooms to cover the bottom of the baking pan)

- 1 tbsp minced garlic

- Salt & pepper to taste

- 2 cups dry white wine or dry vermouth

- ¼ cup fresh chopped parsley

Place rack in center of the oven and preheat to 400 degrees.

Into a lightly oiled baking pan, large enough to hold chicken breasts, arrange mushrooms gill side down. Sprinkle with minced garlic, salt & pepper. Pour wine over the mushrooms. Place chicken breasts, skin side up, over mushrooms and brush with olive oil.

Bake uncovered about 20 minutes until the breasts are golden brown. If the wine has evaporated during the cooking process, add a little more (for those of you who can't tolerate alcohol, keep in mind that it burns off during the cooking process, leaving only the flavor).

Baste the breasts with the pan juices and turn over. Cook until breasts are completed done and springy to the finger, about 15 minutes more.

With a slotted spoon, place the chicken and mushrooms on a platter, mushrooms on the bottom and breasts on top, skin side up. Skim off excess fat and spoon juices over the chicken. Sprinkle with parsley.

Serve with steamed broccoli and boiled new potatoes. (Substitute brown rice for potatoes, if desired)

STIR FRIED SHRIMP AND VEGETABLES

Served over millet, brown rice or quinoa

- 3 tbsp Canola oil
- 1lb. raw medium peeled shrimp
- 2 cups broccoli florets
- 2 cups sliced mushrooms
- 4 scallions, trimmed and chopped
- 2 tbsp Garlic, minced
- 2 tbsp fresh ginger, minced
- 1 cup cold vegetable broth (see recipe above), mixed with 2tbsps, corn starch
- 1 package of organic millet

Into a hot wok or sauté pan, pour oil until just smoking

Add vegetables and stir constantly to cook al dente

Add shrimp and continue to stir until just turning pink

Add broth and cover for a couple of minutes until shrimp is almost done

Uncover and add cornstarch mixture, stir until thickened and turn off heat

Serve over millet cooked according to package instructions

Season to taste with tamari light soy sauce

CHAPTER 13: TASTY ACID REFLUX RECIPES FOR 1 OR 2 WEEKS MUST READ

Note: This dish must be done very quickly, as you don't want to overcook the shrimp or the vegetables. I have chosen Millet because it is an extremely alkaline grain. It is neutral in taste and will absorb the flavors of this dish. You may substitute brown rice instead.

CHAPTER 14:

CREATING YOUR PERSONAL ACID REFLUX RECIPE

Acid reflux is a reality for many, and there are many reasons why it might happen. Though stress can be a problem, often the foods and drinks that people choose are the biggest triggers.

Things like alcohol, soda, spicy foods, fatty foods, and come citrus can bring about a world of pain for some. Some who have GERD-like to put together an acid reflux recipe book to keep track of the foods that don't bother them. Having such a book will make it easier for anyone with this condition to eat the right foods more often.

Before you begin compiling recipes, you should think about how you are going to store them. Your print can them out or write them down, but you may not be able to keep track of them that way. That means you probably aren't going to use them because you can't find them.

A simple three-ring binder is always a great idea, or you can use a box with index cards. These will keep all of your acid reflux recipes in one place.

When it comes to recipes, you might want to consider laminating the pages. This is extra work and an extra expense, but regular paper gets ruined very easily when in the kitchen.

CHAPTER 14: CREATING YOUR PERSONAL ACID REFLUX RECIPE

Laminating will help keep your recipes safe from grease, and they can be wiped off easily if something were to spill.

Finding recipes might be a matter of trial and error, but then there are tons to be found online. A simple search can dig up hundreds. You have to decide what you think sounds good. You can print them out and put them in your binder, or you can write them out on your index cards.

You should start with things that you know you would like, and then slowly add new things you would like to try. GERD sufferers should make sure their recipes are well balanced with proteins and carbs and should be low fat most of the time. Keep that in mind as you browse online.

Don't forget that you can also find great recipes by asking your doctor for recommendations. You can also find recipes by tweaking some of your favorite recipes that give you problems. You can also write them from scratch if you pay attention to what you can eat, and what is known to give you problems.

Things you should avoid would be citrus fruits, milk products (if you suffer from lactose intolerance), spicy foods, many sweets, fatty meats (buy lean cuts), and many forms of white potato.

Though taking the hot spices out of foods might sound like it makes for a bland diet, there are plenty of great herbs and seasonings that won't aggravate acid reflux. It might take you a while to come up with your own collection, but if you add a few new ones a week, your acid reflux recipe book will grow rather quickly.

Though some of the foods that should be avoided bother many, they may not bother you. That is what will make your recipe book unique. If you don't have problems with spicy foods, then, by all means, include them.

There are no hard and fast rules for all people who have GERD. Even more important than what you eat is how you eat.

Remember to eat smaller and more frequent meals, and keep servings small, so your meals are not sitting in your stomach. That might be one of the biggest things to avoid.

CHAPTER 15:

PERMANENT ACID REFLUX CURE

For those unfortunate enough to suffer from regular bouts of heartburn the possibility that there might be a permanent acid reflux cure will seem like the answer to their prayers. But, if you have an open mind and are willing to take an alternative view to solving your problem, your prayers will be answered.

This may seem a fanciful claim as the medical profession tells us that there is no permanent cure for heartburn and that taking some form of drug-based medication is the only way that we can control our problem. It is true that regularly popping those pills has brought that much-needed relief.

So is it possible that there is an alternative way to stop the pain and distress once and for all? The answer is YES and what is more, the cure does not rely on taking any drugs at all. But why are we told that there is no cure for heartburn and acid reflux? Quite simply, if somebody developed a product that could cure our problem, the pharmaceutical industry would lose a fortune in revenue.

Prescribed and over-the-counter medication for heartburn is one of the top money earners in the pharmaceutical industry, so where is the incentive to develop a cure? Cynical, but unfortunately true.

So if the pharmaceutical industry isn't going to provide the cure, where is it going to come from? Well, first of all, we need to understand that the conventional way of treating for acid reflux is to treat the symptoms and mask them by taking a pill.

This is why relief is only temporary. But this ignores a very important fact that acid reflux can be caused by many factors and variables, which include lifestyle, diet, environmental factors, inherited genetic traits, poor digestion, and toxins in the system. Simply dealing with the symptoms of heartburn will never solve the problem.

Doesn't it make sense that if you are going to cure your condition permanently, you must identify, treat and eliminate every one of the factors which are creating the problem? Of course, it does.

Once you have identified those specific factors that are causing your problem you can then set about dealing with them and eliminating them. Eliminate them and the problem will disappear for good.

The most effective way to achieve this is to follow a holistic program of treatment that combines strategic changes to diet and lifestyle with the most appropriate vitamin and herbal supplements. Totally natural and not a drug in sight! Treat the causes and not just the symptoms and you will have found the acid reflux cure which will give you that permanent relief from your heartburn.

All you need is the right guidance. Most conventional treatments for acid reflux and heartburn are temporary because they treat the symptoms and not the root cause of the problem.

So, if you want to successfully and permanently rid yourself of your heartburn then you must identify and address all the factors that contribute to the problem i.e. you must treat it holistically.

Finally, if you found this book useful in anyway, a review on Amazon is always appreciated!

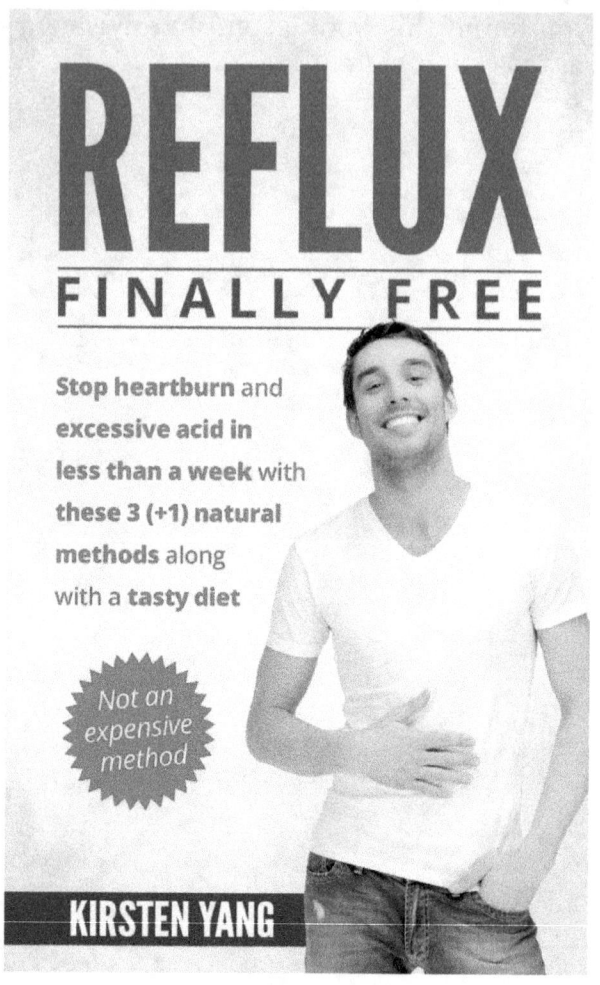

Do You Want to Use Natural Remedies To Cure Acid Reflux!?

Discover 4 Healing Remedies I Personally Used To Get Rid Of Acid Reflux

<u>CLICK HERE AND ADD THE BOOK TO YOUR CART</u>

https://www.amazon.com/Reflux-Finally-heartburn-excessive-natural-ebook/dp/B01N7JPOOD/ref=sr_1_1?s=digital-text&ie=UTF8&qid=1488446561&sr=1-1&keywords=reflux